Exercises for Intending Mindfully: Volume Nine

Mindfulness Practices for Persons with Parkinson's Disease

9/3/2014
Parkinsons Recovery
Robert Rodgers PhD

Exercises for Intending Mindfully
Mindfulness Practices for Persons with Parkinson's Disease
Volume Nine

Contents

The Parkinsons Recovery Mindfulness Series

Realistically speaking, how can the intense level of stress that aggravates the symptoms of Parkinson's disease be calmed? Better yet, how can they be quieted? My research over the past decade reveals that using your mind to drop the stress level down a notch or two always backfires. When you tell yourself:

- *Settle down!*
- *Take it easy!*
- *Stop being so stressed out!*

The stress level ratchets up, not down. Attempts to force the stress and anxiety levels to adjust downward induce an internally generated stress. They pile more stress on top of an excess of stress that already exists. There are certainly a sufficient number of external generators of stress in every one's life. Why infuse more stress that you create yourself, even with the best of intentions?

If the mind is not a useful technique to reduce stress, what is? The most eloquent answer I have for you is to become more mindful of what is experienced in the present moment. Becoming more mindful shifts you into the experience of the "now" which in itself is less stressful (unless you have been kidnapped by terrorists!).

It is stressful to anticipate events you imagine will occur in the future. The events we imagine rarely happen. Does this ring true for you? We all create unnecessary stress in our lives by how and where we focus our thoughts and attention.

It is stressful to agonize over the past. When we think about the past, we are much more likely to think about unpleasant experiences that induce stress. The past event itself was traumatic enough. Yet, we insist on reliving the trauma over and over again through our memories. It seems some of us just can't get enough stress in our lives.

The problem with upping the ante on stress levels is that – as you well know – symptoms of Parkinson's disease become worse. When you are not as stressed, your symptoms are far less problematic.

I have reached one solid conclusion from my ten years of research on Parkinson's disease. Symptoms will drive you crazy when you are stressed and are far less problematic when stress is under control.

Now, if you can't use your mind to become more mindful (which creates added stress in itself) how in the world can you quiet down a frantic lifestyle? I have concluded that the simplest and most effective solution to reducing stress levels is to become more mindful.

The transformation is possible step by step through these simple exercises you can do anywhere, anytime of the day. The Parkinsons Recovery mindfulness exercises are designed to focus your attention on the present moment as attention on either the past or the future is diverted. A renewed focus on the present moment reduces stress levels. Mindfulness is a lifestyle that will reduce stresses in your life if you set the intention to take a mindfulness practice seriously.

I recommend that you practice each of the exercises for a week or longer. Incorporate each practice into your regular routines and habits. Attempts to do all of the exercises simultaneously will likely induce more stress which – obviously – is contrary to the intent of a successful mindfulness program.

Give each exercise a little time and space. Invite the stresses in your life to dissipate. Allow the experience of each practice to engulf you. In so doing, watch the stresses in your life dip down to new lows along with a concurrent relief of any and all symptoms that you have currently been experiencing.

This volume is one out of nine I have developed to support the recovery of persons who currently experience neurological symptoms. A full listing of the Parkinsons Recovery Mindfulness themes follows:

Exercises for Intending Mindfully
Mindfulness Practices for Persons with Parkinson's Disease
Volume Nine

Robert Rodgers, PhD

Parkinsons Recovery

www.parkinsonsrecovery.me

Olympia, Washington

Declaration of Independence

My invitation for you this week is to sign and post a declaration of independence and to do so, if and only if it feels like the right step to take. Many people, myself included, search outside our inner wisdom and intuition for advice and guidance. We take the advice of the experts – persons in white coats or fancy suits or designer dresses. We defer to the judgment of people who have fancy initials beside their name, initials like PhD, MD or ND. When we defer to the judgments of others that contradict our own sense of the right decision to make,

- We give away our power.
- We become dependent on someone else.
- We derail our innate ability to make decisions that are in our best and highest good.

We think:

> *"Surely others are better qualified than I am to know what is in my best interest."*

Yes, it always makes good sense to seek out advice from the experts. To learn what other people recommend is a wise and judicious step to take. Yet, many of us (and I say again myself included) have often wanted someone else to fix us, to make everything all right again. In so doing, we discredit our own inner wisdom and instincts.

It is one thing to say that the body knows how to heal itself. That is certainly a mindful statement. It is also one thing to be sensitive to the signals that our body is always sending to us. Yet, it is easy to slip out of this mindful space and seek relief without checking in with our bodies; without asking whether or not this is in fact what our body truly needs to reverse symptoms.

Your body, my body, any body contains limitless wisdom. We have the power and the ability to know what is in our best interest. Becoming mindful of that wisdom is the key to recovery. Our body is the one and only resource that knows what is best for us. Our body is the one doctor we can always trust.

My invitation then, only if it feels right, is to sign a declaration of independence.

1. **Print it.**
2. **Sign it.**
3. **Post it.**

Declare that you have the inner wisdom that is always present within your body to know what are the best and the right choices to make—options that will help your body come back into full balance and harmony.

Declaration of Independence

In the beginning, one cell was formed inside the womb of our mother that contained the wisdom of all that we are today. The wisdom of one is ten-billion times sevenfold today. We are now equipped with a mind to organize our thoughts, a heart to evaluate them and a voice to express them. At this time and in this hour we declare our minds, hearts and voice to be independent of any and all control over the health and well-being that we have blindly accepted in the past.

We acknowledge the miracle of life itself. We celebrate the ability of our body to rejuvenate despite any and all limitations that we may currently experience. We see the limitless possibility for manifesting any and all dreams for the future. We release any and all limitations for recovery we have imposed on ourselves. We assert our independent right to decide what actions are in our best and highest good.

We understand the conditions that foster neurological imbalances are complex and multifaceted. We ask for and openly receive healing. We pledge from this day forward to listen to the wisdom of our body. We commit to take any

8

and all actions that are required to bring our body back into balance. We agree to transform habits that have been making us ill. We declare independence from the oppressive and dehumanizing claims that recovery is not possible.

We accept full responsibility for the well-being of our own body. We realize it is not constructive to judge any particular treatment option to be superior to any other option or to criticize another person for the options they have chosen to pursue. We know that a therapy or a treatment which helps ourselves may not necessarily be helpful to others and vice versa. By affixing our signatures below, we join with others who honor the power of the body to heal as we restore, rejuvenate and regenerate the inner wisdom of our body to heal.

_____

Signature

Affix your signature to the bottom of this statement. Post it in a public place in your house. Invite others to affix their signatures to the Declaration of Independence. Honor their decision to sign or not to sign. By affixing your signature to this Declaration, you have become more mindful of the power of the body to heal itself.

Deeper Meaning Behind a Declaration of Independence

Permit me to explain the connection between the Declaration of Independence that you were invited to sign and post this week and the American Declaration of Independence that was signed by the founding fathers in 1776.

My great, great, great grandfather was named David Rush. David Rush was a cousin of one of the signers of the Declaration of Independence, Benjamin Rush. In the early years of his life Benjamin Rush visited England and was awed by the regality of the Crown. He saw no more awesome heights to aspire to than to become a member of the royal court. He was convinced that the British way of life was a way of life to be coveted, admired and honored.

Soon after his trip Benjamin Rush changed his mind. As it turned out there was significant oppression by the British toward the Americans with regard to taxation and other matters. The British held the attitude that the Americans were slaves and servants of the British. The Americans were a lower class to be put into the closet and quieted, even if it meant military action was necessary and needed. Sounds to me like a familiar theme today as expressed in America.

The Americans stepped forward in 1776 and declared their independence. They began to make strong statements about their right to live their life the way they wanted to live it – to earn a living without the encumbrances of having a higher power (like a King) or authority (like the military) ordering them what to do and how to do it.

What then is the connection between the American Declaration of Independence and the Declaration of Independence that I invited you to sign and post this week? I have heard too many horrifying stories of the response people have had to being told that they have been diagnosed with Parkinson's disease. It is a horrible experience for most persons. Being "diagnosed" means they will eventually lose their freedom – or at least that is the first impression. Words that are spoken by those who convey the diagnosis have a devastating impact. The condition is "degenerative." It is "progressive." Treatments can only slow the "progression." How depressing can you get!

A diagnosis is only the opinion of one person. Other people may well have different opinions. My research shows that a vast majority of people who have been diagnosed with Parkinson's disease do not have it! They have some other combination of problems and imbalances that have been pestering the sensitive neurological system such as toxins, infections and traumas.

I see a profound connection between being told of a diagnosis of Parkinson's disease and the events of the British oppressing the spirit and the life force and the dreams of the American people in the 1700's. It is really the same in my book of analogies.

Are we going to accede to the authority of an "other", whatever that "other" might be – whether a country or a person regardless of their qualifications or rank? Are we willing to accept the edicts of a King of England simply because they are a King?

Americans over two centuries ago were not. When it comes to any diagnosis – and in this case Parkinson's disease – I believe it is wise to step forward and assert our independence.

Our body does have the wisdom and the knowledge to heal all imbalances. The natural condition of the body is to be in harmony, not disharmony. Once we begin to be mindful of the signals our body gives to us, once we honor the limitless knowledge and wisdom that is contained within our body, we accelerate our ability to reverse symptoms of Parkinson's disease.

Of course it is important to seek advice from others, whether they be physical therapists, chiropractors, medical doctors, naturopath doctors, researchers, neuro-feedback practitioners, bio-acoustic practitioners, Feldenkrais practitioners, cranial-sacral practitioners,

Bowen practitioners, acupuncturists, herbalists, masters of tai chi and Qigong, spiritual masters - the list is endless. Of course it is important to study research and consider options.

But in the end, the final decision resides with us. We have the power to heal. It is now time to be mindful of that power, to actualize that power, to turn the switch in our thinking, the switch that says wrongly, falsely and harmfully that Parkinson's is a degenerative condition.

Of course medicines may be needed or required. Of course supplements may be needed or required. Perhaps surgeries will be facilitative. Nothing that I have argued here suggests that there is any single therapy or option or approach that is superior to another.

Your body is truly a unique and sacred vessel. The imbalances are unique to you as a person. There is no one like you. Dig deeply and you will begin to identify the options that need to be pursued for becoming symptom-free.

If you have decided to sign and post the Declaration of Independence, you are warmly and cordially invited to recruit others to do the same. No diagnosis of Parkinson's disease is required or necessary. You see, the Declaration of Independence pertains to each and every individual who occupies a body, a condition that we all meet.

May we join together as a community of individuals who are committed in our hearts, minds and souls to the idea that we have limitless wisdom that is contained within us. We have the ability to make good decisions.

- Acknowledge that wisdom now.
- Accept that power now.
- Actualize your life force now.
- Celebrate each and every moment of your recovery as it unfolds ever so gently and effortlessly.

Look forward to the opportunity to celebrate a life that affords endless opportunities for abundance, health, wealth and all treasures that your heart desires.

Relationship With Time

What is your relationship with time? Is it a good one? Is it positive? Or, is your relationship with time stressed? Are you traumatized each time you have an appointment?

- *Are you a person who is always early?*
- *Are you a person who is always on time?*
- *Are you a person who is consistently and habitually always late?*

What is your orientation and perception of time? It is that orientation and perception that can potentially create significant stress or significantly reduce stress.

The invitation and challenge I have for you this week is to be mindful about your own thoughts and reactions to time. I have three challenges, three invitations for you. The first invitation is to set your intention to be particularly early to an appointment that you have this week. This might be your regular routine, but please be early anyway. Access how you feel about being early.

1. *Does it feel good?*
2. *Does it feel bad?*
3. *What are your thoughts?*

The second invitation is to – as best as possible – plan out your day so that you are precisely on time to an

15

appointment. Arrive not a minute early or a minute late. Then as before, check in to see how you feel about being precisely on time.

1. *Does it feel good?*
2. *Does it feel bad?*
3. *What are your thoughts?*

Finally, the third invitation (you probably see this one coming) is to be intentionally late by 10 or 15 minutes to an appointment that you have scheduled this week. Access for yourself your own feelings and reactions to what that experience means for you.

1. *Does it feel good?*
2. *Does it feel bad?*
3. *What are your thoughts**?*

The challenge of the week is to systematically and mindfully assess your own personal reactions to what it means to be on time. I am fully aware that some of you are habitually early, some of you are habitually always on time and some of you are habitually late. It is very possible that any one of the three routines of habit (being either early, on time or late) may create significant stress for you. If you are unable to accept any one of these three challenges, ask yourself:

How does it feel to refuse the challenge?

16

If you are up to it this week accept all three challenges. Assess your personal reactions and feelings in the moment. This is what becoming more mindful is all about.

Be sure to have fun with this one. You will find it will be an interesting experience that offers the promise of revealing ways that you have been creating stress unnecessarily. Have a marvelous week as you enjoy implementing the three mindfulness challenges.

Deeper Meaning Behind Your Relationship to Time

While I focused the three challenges of this week on our orientation to time by intentionally being early, on intentionally being exactly on time and intentionally being late - the three challenges actually have little to do with time itself. They have everything to do with our mind states, our habits and our thought patterns. Our relationship to time is wrapped up in the state of our ego which does not always have our best interest at heart.

Time is actually irrelevant. Why? We are always mindful when live in the present moment. Time has no meaning whatsoever other than the meaning we ourselves attribute to it.

If we habitually find that we always are late to appointments, we may be carrying certain thought forms like,

- *"I'm a very busy person. I don't have time to wait around for other people to arrive to the meeting."*
- *"I'm a very important person so in order to be able to assert my importance I will arrive late to every meeting that I actually attend. I want everyone to see that I am important. I cannot attend any meeting that happens to arbitrarily start at a very specific time."*

Perhaps you are a person who is routinely and habitually always on time to appointments. What are the feelings and thought processes driving this habit? Is it perhaps because you like to be seen as:

- *A person who is a perfectionist?*
- *A person who is reliable?*
- *A person who is trustworthy?*
- *A person who cares about others so you do not want them to be waiting around just for you?*
- *A person who wants to be precisely on time because you cannot tolerate the anxiety that is associated with being early or late?*

Or perhaps you are person who is routinely and habitually early to all appointments. Is it perhaps because you:

- *Do not want to be seen if you come late?*
- *Do not want to be judged as unreliable?*
- *Do not want to waste other people's time because they are more important than you?*

Of course I could go on and on with many different rationales and thoughts that float through our minds whether we are early, on time or late. Regardless of the thought, it certainly does not serve our best and highest good.

When it comes to reducing stress, the ideal strategy is to give yourself plenty of opportunity to get wherever it is that you need to get. Plan ahead even if it means you may be a bit early to appointments. This way, there is no stress involved in worrying about whether or not you might be late – if in fact being late is a worry you find that you oftentimes have.

The challenge this week is to evaluate and to assess your relationship with what it means to be "on time" and to consider the possibility of loosening the link between when you arrive and when you are planning on arriving to your appointments. This will enable you to be more in the moment, more mindful of each and every experience that you are having in the "now".

When we are focused on time we are always thinking about the future. In other words, we are focused on arriving at a location at a future point in time. That, as it turns out, is not being mindful.

Set a new habit so that you give yourself plenty of time.

- *Start preparing to leave early.*
- *Slow everything down.*
- *Relish the pleasure of dressing to get ready.*
- *Hear the sound of your footsteps.*
- *Enjoy the journey as you enter into your car or bus or train or plane.*

Moreover, take in the full experience of each step of the journey to wherever it is that you are going. Drop all worries about being on time or about being late. Such worries only cause unnecessary stress.

Continue if you so choose a self-examination of your orientation to time. Cast aside any bad attitudes you may hold. Allow yourself to become fully and completely focused on the present moment (regardless of whether you are early, on time or late to appointments!).

- This is the place you will derive limitless pleasure.
- This is the place where stress has no opportunity to enter into the tissues of your body.
- This is the place that requires no travel.
- You are always there.

How much time did you allocate today to read this follow-up to the mindfulness challenge about time? Are you behind time now? Will you now be unable to accomplish everything on your daily plan of activities? Did it take you longer than you had planned to read this section? Or, was there no anticipation or plan for the day?

You see, time is simply whatever we make it out to be. Make time your ally not your enemy.

Desires

The mindfulness invitation this week is to become – as often as possible throughout the day – aware of what you really desire.

- *Do you desire sweets in the moment, perhaps a piece of chocolate or pie?*
- *Do you desire caffeine?*
- *Do you desire sleep?*
- *Do you desire a shopping trip?*
- *Do you desire fast food?*
- *Do you desire companionship?*
- *Do you desire a partner that you perhaps currently do not have?*
- *Do you desire to hang out with friends?*

Desires arise continuously throughout each day. We often think of desires as being only in two categories: sex and food. But desires often consume the choices that we make. The challenge for the week is to become aware of what you desire in the moment, minute by minute, hour by hour. Have a delightful time as you become more aware of what you desire from moment to moment.

Deeper Meaning Behind Desires

What is the deeper meaning behind becoming aware of what you desire moment by moment throughout the day? Desires are what charge us up.

- *They give us an infusion of energy. It is as if we are getting an adrenaline shot.*
- *They help us feel alive.*
- *They help us feel as though we are living a full and vibrant life.*

Take for example the experience of desiring a car. When we desire a car we begin to look around and search for a vehicle that is perfectly suited for us, our needs and the needs of our family.

- *We visit lots that have cars for sale.*
- *We talk to friends.*
- *We notice cars on the highway*
- *We evaluate cars parked on downtown streets.*
- *We form judgments about which cars we really like and those we do not like.*
- *We calculate the extent to which we can afford or not afford the car we really desire.*

The decision over buying a car consumes our thoughts – at least temporarily. That desire fills our spirit and our mind with an infusion of energy. This is a good thing.

The difficulty is that we become addicted to certain patterns of behavior that are guaranteed to deliver an instant rush of energy. This, of course, is a well-known habitual pattern for anyone who is an addict which includes pretty much everyone. We are all addicted to some particular type of behaviors. Some habitual behaviors are far, far more harmful to our bodies than others.

In terms of individuals who currently experience the symptoms of Parkinson's, there is no doubt that foods can have a dramatic impact on health and wellness. Certain foods help relieve symptoms. Other foods aggravate symptoms. The connection is immediate. This means of course that if you have a persistent nag to eat certain foods that you know are not in your best and highest good, you will suffer the consequences.

The road to recovery requires that we become more aware of the consequences of insisting that our desires always be fulfilled. Is a desire something that is healthy and needs to be pursued vigorously? Or, is it something that is not in our best and highest good?

24

Perhaps yesterday morning you thought to yourself,

> *"Oh, I know I really need to go out and get my regular exercise today."*

Then you think,

> *"But wouldn't it be nice to cuddle up, have a nice pot of tea and watch that show that I've been wishing to watch?"*

It may be that watching that show cuddled up on a couch is precisely what it is that you and your body need in the moment, but it is also possible that this desire is undermining your own best and highest good. It may be that the better choice in the moment is to jump start your body with exercise rather than choosing stagnation.

Becoming aware of our desires becomes an exercise of realizing how much our desires control our choices. The real question turns on whether or not we desire something or need something. Desires piggyback on past experiences that offer us instant energetic charges. Needs are something that arise from a much deeper place.

We remember what it was like to eat that delicious chocolate cake. We think to ourselves,

"If I have that chocolate now I am going to get that same incredible surge of pleasure and energy; so I'm going to do it right now."

It is possible to get those surges of energy in other healthy ways as we become much more mindful, moment to moment of the choices that we make and the desires that arise. Desires will always consume our choices if we let them. Unhealthy desires will maintain our body in a continual state of imbalance and illness. The trick of reversing neurological symptoms is to act on healthy desires and reject the unhealthy ones.

Become, then, continuously aware over the next several days of what you desire. Know that what you desire may in fact be incredibly healthy for you and your body, family and friends. This choice affords the opportunity to reverse symptoms.

It is also possible that what you desire in the moment is in fact just the reverse. It is obviously not in your best and highest good. Acting on unhealthy desires aggravates symptoms, causes depression and aggravates symptoms.

Becoming more aware of what you desire is 90% of what you need to know to make informed and healthy choices for yourself and your future. May you have a delightful week as you monitor the meaning and consequence of what it is that, in fact, you desire moment to moment.

26

Procrastination

This exercise invites you to become attentive and might I say, mindful of all of the ways that you procrastinate. Permit me be clear however. When I say procrastinate I am really referring to the little things, to the small stuff. We all procrastinate on big decisions in our lives, decisions like

- *Should I marry this person or not?*
- *Should I have a child or not?*
- *Should I move to North Dakota or not?*
- *Should I quit my job or keep my job?*

These are big decisions that require thought and some intuitive instincts about what is right for you and your family that need to incubate, evolve and take shape over time. With time and a little incubation, the big decisions become clearer.

The procrastination that I am referring to is procrastinating over the small things. We are certainly different people so I am quite sure my list of how I procrastinate will differ from yours. However, permit me to offer a few possibilities by way of providing an insight into exactly what I am getting at here. Here are a few of the ways that I procrastinate.

27

- *Do you procrastinate when the mail is received? "Oh, I'll just put that aside. I don't really have time to shift through the mail right now."*

- *Do you procrastinate when you receive an e-mail from a close friend that requires a response? "Well, that's not what I planned to do right now so I'm not going to respond to that e-mail at this very moment."*

- *Do you procrastinate when you pay a bill that arrives in the snail mail? "Oh, let me open up the bill, see what it is. Oh wow, that's a little more than I expected. Let me just put that away in my little drawer where I keep my bills. I'll attend to paying this one at a later point this particular month."*

- *Do you procrastinate over washing the dishes when the dishes are dirty? "Oh – I did not use one of those dirty dishes. Let them wash them all."*

- *Do you procrastinate over buying a present for a relative whose birthday is coming up next week and you think, "Today is the day I really should buy them a birthday present. Today really is not too soon, but wait a minute, today was not the day that I planned on doing that so I'll have to defer that activity until tomorrow."*

28

- *Do you procrastinate when you think to yourself, "I really would like to talk to my son, my daughter, my mother, my father, my uncle, my aunt, my grandfather, my grandmother" – you know, the people who are important to us. Do you think, "Oh I really ought to call them today" and then the next thought is, "Oh no, no, no, I really don't have time. That call will take some time and, as I think about the day that I have planned there's not enough time."*

- *Do you procrastinate when the phone rings and you hear a message on your phone answering machine. You say to yourself, "That's important for me to answer but I really don't feel up to talking with that person right now. I'll answer that call later today or well, maybe I'll put it off until tomorrow."*

- *Do you procrastinate when you think to yourself, "During the day I need to go out and get all of the trash in the trash bin for the trash person to pick up who is coming tomorrow. I need to do that right now because later on tonight it really might be too dark for me to see and it may be that it will be raining. But it will probably not rain tonight so I will just wait until later"*

29

I obviously could go on and on with a list of the ways that I procrastinate. Are some of these ways that you procrastinate too? I will cut off my list of the many ways I procrastinate (which it would fill up a 400 page book if I continued).

For the next several days be mindful about all of the many ways that you set aside the small stuff that needs to be taken care of; those minor little tasks that all the sudden come up.

- You know the task needs to be done at some point.
- You know you need to do at some point.
- But when?

You simply put the small tasks aside routinely for what seems to be good reasons.

How do you procrastinate?

1. Reflect.
2. Become aware.
3. Acknowledge when you procrastinate.
4. Track every little small task you aside.

If you want to get really serious about this exercise, record all of the ways you put off doing the small stuff and little tasks during the day.

Implications of Procrastination

How long has your list of procrastination opportunities become? When I started tracking the ways that I procrastinate, my list was amazingly long. I surprised myself by the number of times every day that I put a small task aside to be replaced by doing something that I thought was more important.

This exercise has helped me make important changes to the choices I make about the small stuff every day. The small stuff adds up. As a result of the changes I have made to attending to the small stuff, I have become much more mindful and less stressed. This, my friends, is what a successful mindfulness practice can achieve for us all.

Here is what I discovered when I really began to watch and observe my behavior. Yes, I put aside many, many small tasks. What were the consequences of that? The first major consequence was that every day I would have at least two hours (if not three hours) of thoughts that rattled through my mind about all of those unfinished tasks that I needed to remind myself to be sure and complete. I make no overstatement here. I was occupying a lot of my brain capacity to making sure I remembered to get back to all of those small tasks that I had so casually set aside the day before (or month before for that matter).

My brain was always filled to the brim with a long list of unfinished tasks that needed to be completed.

What do these thoughts sound like if I were to voice them to you now? I would be thinking to myself,

> *"Oh yeah, that's right I've got to write that letter to Betty that I promised that I would write."*

> *"That's right, I've got to buy that present for a friend and that's going to be due in a couple of weeks so I have to be sure and get that done."*

> *"There are four or five emails I didn't respond to last week. I can't remember quite what they were but I'm sure I've got to do that at least sometime in the next couple of days. Yea, they are probably waiting for a reply – well of course I just don't have time right now to get back to them. It will probably take me 10 or 15 minutes to even find their emails. I don't have enough time now to look back in my emails from a couple of weeks ago to find who it was that wrote me and what it was they wanted. All of that is just too much work for me to do right now."*

> *"And yeah, that bill, I know that bill for the internet is due. If they shut my internet down I'm really shut down for good so let me think about it. Yeah. That is one I really ought to do right now but I really*

don't want to do it. I hate to pay bills but I'm going to go find that internet bill right now. It is probably back in that box where I put all the bills."

So what do I do? I march back to the box. I'm very proud of myself because I am actually attending to something I know I have to do. I can't put off any longer. And guess what? I can't find the bill. The bill is not in the box. So I say to myself,

"But I've really got to pay this bill now. I think it's due today or at least maybe tomorrow so I've got to pay it today or else I'll have to pay the late fee and my internet might actually be shut down."

What then happens? We're talking 15, 20 minutes, 30 minutes – sometimes an hour – I have to launch a search. I begin to think,

"Let's see, when did that bill come in? That was two weeks ago and, okay, I went to the mailbox, or was that Deborah? I can't quite remember that. Maybe I did go to the mailbox and I picked up the mail and then I came in the house and where was I when I looked at the mail?

Let's see, well maybe I left it in the car, that's possible. Well let me get the keys to the car, I'll go out to the car right now. I will look in the car and see if the bill is in the car. Maybe it is in the car."

33

I go out to the car. The bill is not in the car.

> *"Okay, that didn't work, let me go back in the house. Where was I when I saw the bill? I remember opening the bill, I remember about how much it was, so where did I open up the bill?"*

Okay, I could go on and on and explain to you the process of what I encounter when I have these types of experiences (and there have been many). My frustration level begins to get higher and higher and higher because I can't find the bill. I know it needs to be paid but I simply can't get the task done.

I come to a decision point after 45 minutes of looking.

1. Do I just give up?
2. Do I find a different way to pay the bill, like maybe going to the company itself?
3. Do I go online and see if I can find the invoice (although I don't even know how to do that)?
4. Do I just say, "I won't bother paying the bill this time? They'll send me another one, I'll have a late fee, what does it matter?"

How do I solve the problem? In other words it engages a whole sequence of activities and challenges that were entirely unnecessary. This is only one small example. It is often the case that when I get ready to do something that I know has to be done, I can't find the materials that I need in order to complete the task.

What then is the change that I made in my life? It has been a gradual change but what I decided to do is this: When the small little tasks were in my face I started acknowledging when I procrastinated (for, of course, a presumably very smart and rational reason). It's pretty easy to do. It's not as if there's any secret to when you procrastinate, the thought is,

> *"Oh, I can't do that right now I don't have enough time."*

Or a favorite of mine is,

> *"I don't want to do that right now. I've done 10 tasks that I really didn't want to do today but I had to do. If I do this one it will be number eleven. I'm sorry. I'm not going to do the 11th task. That's just over the board for me. I'm going to go do something that I want to do!"*

That's usually my rationale. Of course the difficulty as it turns out, since I use the rationale so often --

> *"I don't have time to do it right now."*

The little small tasks that I put aside begin to mount up one on top of another on top of another. Soon I have 20,

25, 30 if not 40 undone tasks in the queue, all of which are splattered in different compartments of my memory. To complete any these unfinished tasks I have to go back in time and reconstruct what it was that I needed to do (or promised to do). It takes me four, five or ten times longer to do the task than it would have taken had I simply done the task when it first came to my attention.

I then made a decision when I recognized all the ways that I procrastinated that I would change my habitual way of behaving. When the little stuff needs to be done and I hear myself saying,

> *"I'm going to put that aside."*

I stop. I take a breath. I say,

> *"Whoa! Hold on just a minute! Let's do that little task right now."*

Yes, it does take a little time if I have to pay a bill or respond to an email. But then, the task is done. I have finished it!

When I need to respond to a question in an email, research is often required which is why I always set the task aside in the past. Writing up a response may take 30 minutes or longer. But, when I set aside the task, it takes twice as long to respond. Why? It takes me 30 minutes to find the question in my saved emails.

Doing the task in the moment when it comes up is much more efficient for me. It also feels a whole lot better when I complete the task when the email comes through than when I set the task aside.

Don't get me wrong. I do put things aside every once in a while. I often get questions that I literally do not know the answer to. Research is required that takes several hours if not longer. I may not have enough time to do that work in the moment. I do not attend to every task immediately. Some tasks really do take quite a bit of time to complete. But, when somebody asks me to do something, I make every effort to do it immediately.

People who ask for information need it now. I now offer a response which is a start at solving their problem. I respond when I get the question. This way I do not have to dig back in my emails to find the question that was asked. What exactly did that person ask me? It winds up being so much more time-consuming. It eats up my energy to go back and do the job if it sits on the shelf for a day or two days or three weeks or four weeks. Attending the tasks as they come through is a healing and energizing experience.

The other benefit for me personally has been that it eliminates the problem of stuck energy. When we put things aside we create clogs in our energetic system. Setting tasks aside drains our life force. Clogs and blocks in our energetic system slow everything down. There is no flow. No life force is present. Becoming less of a procrastinator creates more flow.

We are not able to manifest abundance or health or wellness if our "to do lists" are dozens of pages long. The flow in my life is much better now that I have begun to attend to the little stuff in a timely fashion.

Why not attend to the small stuff when it comes up rather than putting it off? For all of those little tasks that you tend to put aside – perhaps the phone calls that you know you need to make – make them now! You don't have to talk a long time. You can simply tell the person,

> *"I just wanted to touch base and say hi, how are you; and by the way I've got an appointment in 15 minutes, I can't talk long."*

That response is perfectly acceptable and it finishes that particular obligation.

Experiment with doing little tasks as they come up. Do not put off doing the little stuff when it comes across your desk or through your computer, phone, friends, family and neighbors.

Of course you may choose to say "No" to a request. This is a smart way to clear out unfinished business before it begins to clutter up your thoughts. Simply make your position clear:

- *No, I'm not going to do that.*
- *No, I'm not going to attend that meeting.*
- *No, I'm not going to meet that appointment. I've just decided it's not something that I can do right now."*

That clears everything up. You have decided. This is so much better than putting aside the decision ...

- *Maybe I should do that...*
- *Maybe I should go to that meeting ...*
- *Maybe I should have an appointment with that person...*

Instead of juggling conflicting and troublesome thoughts about what to do, you stop and say,

"What do I really need to do for myself?"

You make a decision. You respond to the person. It is done. It is complete. There is closure. There is no more pontificating or worrying or agonizing over what it is that you should do or need to do.

Again I want to say for me, working on the various ways that I procrastinate has been life-changing. The flow is much better in my life today than it was a year ago because I now act on all the small stuff. Paying attention to the small stuff really does make a big difference.

I invite you to launch this particular challenge for longer than a week. See how it goes for you. This may be the first week of engaging new habits that pave the road to recovery with:

- More flow
- More abundance
- More health
- More wellness
- More joy

When the above energies are activated, stress takes a back seat to the intention to reverse any and all symptoms associated with a diagnosis of Parkinson's disease.

Jump Start Your Day

My Mindfulness Challenge for you this week will consume at most ten seconds each day. The exciting news I have for you is that it will transform your day and your week if you actually do what I am about to suggest that you do.

The minute that you become conscious in the morning after sleeping through the night, the first thought that you have needs to be the following;

"Today will be a magnificent day."

You might want to change that adjective from day to day or simply say whatever comes to mind since you are just coming into consciousness from a deep sleep. When waking the first thing in the morning it can be a bit difficult to think clearly. The statement might be for example:

"Today will be a spectacular day." or

"Today will be a stupendous day." or

"Today will be a terrific day." or

"Today will be an amazing day."

You get the point. Whatever adjective comes to mind when you wake up in the morning, state that magnificent expectation as your first thought of the day. You can say it out loud or think it.

This challenge is actually difficult, not because it consumes time, but because it is very difficult to remember to start your day in a new way as you are waking up. Do your best to remember to state the affirmation each morning when you wake up. If you are up after five minutes, ten minutes or even an hour and you think to yourself,

"Whoops, I forgot to state my affirmation today"

You can still do it even if an hour has passed. Best however if the minute you come to consciousness, before any other thought creeps through your consciousness, to state the affirmation either out loud or silently,

"Today will be a magnificent day."

"Today will be a spectacular day."

Of course because you are still half asleep you are probably not going to make your affirmation with much enthusiasm. Offer the affirmation as best you can.

To summarize, the challenge of the week is - before any other thoughts creep into your consciousness as you awake in the morning – state in your thoughts or out loud your positive expectation for the day about to be lived.

Deeper Implications Behind How You Start Your Day

I have actually been working with this particular Mindfulness Challenge for some time now. My personal experience has been that I am likely to forget to do it. Remembering is my biggest challenge.

When I do remember to make the statement when I wake up, my day turns out to be magnificent, spectacular, stupendous, terrific and even amazing. It is really a magical formula for how to set a positive template for the upcoming day. Planting the seed of a positive intention for the day makes all the difference in the world.

My experience has been that if I don't remember to assert a positive expectation as my first thought, my thinking tends to rattle around in a somewhat negative vein. As I begin to get up out of the bed I may be thinking to myself,

> *"Oh my goodness, looks like it's raining again today."*

That is not a positive thought or a positive statement. Or, as I'm getting up I might be thinking,

> *"Boy, I sure have an achy back! My goodness, what did I do last night?"*

Or, I might think to myself,

"That was sure a long, scary nightmare that I had last night; oh yuck!"

These thoughts may sound familiar to you or not – but we all certainly begin our day with thoughts that are often negative. I have actually noticed as I have become more mindful about my first thought of the day that my first thoughts tend to be much more negative than positive.

My experience has also been that when I remember to make my affirmation at the outset of the day, I set in motion a positive expectation. My thoughts all of a sudden spin the entire day in a positive direction. I'm thinking positively rather than negatively from the get--go. I have noticed a huge difference in how my day unfolds.

My experience has little to do with what is happening to me as a result of circumstances outside my control. The difference is in the way that I respond to those circumstances; even if when I have to confront an pleasant circumstance or encounter that is unexpected. I take the blows in stride, shake them off and move forward to more positive experiences.

As you are well aware, our thoughts have a profound impact on our lives. Start each of your days with a positive thought. There is power in setting a positive expectation at the get go. Avoid the rattle-trap of negativity which will always drag you down into the gutter.

44

Give this challenge a chance, not just this week but for subsequent weeks. I say again I've been working on this now for some time and I am quite pleased with the outcome from meeting the challenge. It is difficult however to break the habit of starting out the day in a fit of negativity.

It is simple to make a positive affirmation at the beginning of the day. It takes at most ten seconds. The real challenge is to remember doing it. Perhaps I have an unconscious voice deep inside that insists every day be horrible. I now prefer to override that voice.

May each day of this week and the rest of the weeks of the year be spectacular, magnificent and amazing as you start each day the right way.

Has your work on these exercises been stress free? Has it been helpful in reducing your symptoms? I certainly hope so! This is the primary reason I developed the mindfulness exercises in the first place.

If you struggled with pacing out these mindfulness exercises so as not to induce more stress, there are several Parkinsons Recovery programs that might help expedite your recovery. My Parkinsons Recovery Mindfulness Program sends the mindfulness exercises in an email to you each and every week. The initial exercise is sent to your email address on day one of the week and the deeper implications are sent four days later. The Parkinsons Recovery Mindfulness Program takes one full year to complete as each exercise is introduced one week at a time. For more information visit:

www.stress.parkinsonsrecovery.com

Parkinsons Recovery Memberships involve a variety of support websites that are essential to recovery. A difference mindfulness exercise is posted each week. For more information on Parkinsons Recovery memberships visit:

www.parkinsonsrecovery.org

Of course, the approach that works for many people is to purchase a single volume of the Parkinsons Recovery

Mindfulness program at a time as you have already done! See the introduction for a listing of all nine Parkinsons Recovery Mindfulness volumes.

Thank you for Your Support

On behalf of the thousands of followers of Parkinsons Recovery, I want to thank you for your purchase of this booklet. One hundred percent (100%) of the profits purchases of my books and programs help subsidize the many free services I offer through Parkinsons Recovery -

www.parkinsonsrecovery.com

For information about other products, services and programs visit -

www.parkinsonsrecovery.me